LOSE WEIGHT FEEL GREAT

Kevin Given

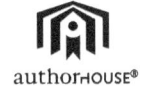

authorHOUSE®

AuthorHouse™
1663 Liberty Drive, Suite 200
Bloomington, IN 47403
www.authorhouse.com
Phone: 1-800-839-8640

First published by AuthorHouse 4/7/2009

ISBN: 978-1-4389-6052-4 (sc)

Printed in the United States of America
Bloomington, Indiana

This book is printed on acid-free paper.

CONTENTS

1) AMERICA'S WEIGHT PROBLEM

I was in the majority; now I'm in the minority, and I'm glad! This country has an increasing battle of the bulge; a weight problem to the point where almost 65 percent of adult Americans are overweight with a body mass index (BMI) above 20.0, and more than a quarter surpass 30.0. That is downright obese!

In 1962, statistics showed that America's population was about 13 percent overweight; by 1980 it had gone up to 15 percent, by 1994 it was 23 percent, and by 2000 it had reached 31 percent. Today it's close to 65 percent. America has truly gone from eating to live to living to eat (research done by the Centers for Disease Control). According to the surgeon general's report, obesity claims the lives of 300,000 per year and it's not getting any better! The amount of overweight kids has more than tripled!

This growth in weight gain is parallel to the growth of fast food! As our pace becomes more hectic and we have less free time, it becomes easier to hit a drive-thru than to take the time and prepare a healthy meal.

3.8 Million Americans carry over 300 lbs

In 1962, there were only a handful of fast food restaurants in this country! By 2000, there were literally thousands operating and serving fatty fried foods to millions of Americans each day!

The film *Supersize Me* chronicles a month in the life of Morgan Spurlock, who went on a complete McDonald's diet for thirty days. Spurlock ate nothing but McDonald's food during that time, for breakfast, lunch, and dinner. He of course endangered his health along the way.

Spurlock ingested 5,000 calories each day. When he started his experiment his weight was around 185 lbs (at 6'2"). By the end of that month, Spurlock had gained 24.5 lbs. It would take him fourteen months to lose it.

Apparently Spurlock was trying to make a point about fast food. He was inspired to do this experiment by a court case where two girls sued McDonald's, claiming that their food made them fat! They lost! All I have to say about that is DUH! For the record, I'm glad that McDonald's won that case!

Nobody forces anybody to eat at McDonald's; you do so of your own free will. You can go wherever you want and eat whatever you want, whether it's good for you or not. That's the beauty of living in a free country, and if you don't know by now that Big Macs are bad for you, then who could tell you?

Closing fast food restaurants by force will not solve the nation's obesity problem, and even if you're out with your own little clique and they decide to stop at McDonalds to eat, no one forces you to eat a Big Mac or a Quarter Pounder. You could always get a salad or a grilled chicken wrap or even a yogurt! Suing fast food restaurants is not the answer.

I do not believe in having Uncle Sam baby-sit us. People have to take the initiative and start eating right on their own.

400,000, mostly men, top the 400-lb limit!

Prohibition didn't stop the alcoholic from getting his booze, and shutting down fast food restaurants won't stop the junk food junkie from getting his Big Mac!

So what did Spurlock accomplish? Well, he made himself sick! That's about the supersize of it! Even though I think McDonald's should have won that court case, I still feel that it's time we as a nation did something to curb the obesity problem in America. Proper education and nutrition programs are the answer, not shutting down fast food restaurants by force or putting a legal ban on trans fat, as Governor Schwarzenegger has done here in sunny California. To sum it up, I appreciate Mr. Spurlock trying to bring about a public awareness to a serious problem, but I don't think that going after fast food restaurants is the answer.

How bad is the problem? We've already seen that the percentage of overweight people has gone from 13 percent in 1962 to almost 65 percent today! That's more than a 50 percent gain in overweight people in today's world from what it was in our parents' generation. We should also mention that the number of overweight children has tripled! A recent *Time* magazine article shed some light on the problem among our youth. Let's look at what *Time* had to say about this problem (*Time* magazine June 23, 2008).

We looked at the adult population from 1962 to the present day according to the CDC (Centers for Disease Control); now let's look at those who are under eighteen. According to the *Journal of the American Medical Association*, the number of six- to eleven-year-olds who were overweight in 2004 was 19 percent; in 1971 it was only 4 percent. A full 32 percent of all American kids are overweight, and 90 percent of those have at least one avoidable risk factor for heart disease! These are scary numbers, and today's kids, of course, are tomorrow's adults! If the problem persists then the next generation could see close to 80 percent of Americans with a weight problem. By 2059, some estimate, all Americans could be overweight! I have made it my goal to see the statistics for obesity in this nation begin to reduce in number within the next five years! This problem is reaching epidemic levels!

The Pixar film *Wall-E* received some flak for depicting human beings of the future as being soft and obese. This criticism is unjust given today's statistics that we have just looked at! The film is simply mirroring a trend in today's society.

Critics are so sensitive when a film deals with a legitimate problem in a realistic manner. We don't want to face the fact that we have a legitimate problem, so the answer for these critics is to simply ignore it! Do they feel that the problem is just going to go away? That solution didn't work for the budget deficit, nor will it work for America's weight problem.

The best Hollywood productions enlighten us while they entertain us! I'm sure that the people involved with making *Wall-E* are not simply trying to poke fun at obese Americans but also want to make us aware of a growing trend, I'm also sure that someone involved with the production of that film is aware of the statistics that we have just looked at.

To try to censor a filmmaker saying what he or she feels needs to be said is wrong! The same goes for a novelist or a screenwriter. I want to put my political two cents in right here. And then I'll get back on track with weight loss!

Any artist should be allowed to create, whether it's a book or film, what he or she feels they should create! It is wrong to put out a reward for the heads of the Salman Rushdies of the world.

Michael Moore's film *Fahrenheit 911* was nothing more than an attack on President Bush in an effort to unseat him; one need only watch the counter-film, *Fahrenhype 911*, to see where Michael Moore manipulated the facts to influence people.

If you do not like President Bush, that's your business and I'm not going to sing the praises of George Bush or condemn the man in this book. We all have our own political views, and I'm not going to preach mine to you here, but the point that needs to be made is that whether you like President Bush or not, you should not misrepresent what he believes, if you practice ethical journalism. Granted, Michael Moore is not a journalist, but should his film have garnered media praise just because the president is not high in popularity polls?

The mainstream media can and should produce whatever it wants, but I believe that journalists have a responsibility to be fair and unbiased in how they report. Are mainstream journalists fair when they report on the president? Look at how they reported his views on stem cell research and you tell me.

Michael Moore seems to be God to liberals and Satan to conservatives. Someone who is a far-left-leaning Democrat will like his film, and someone who is a far-right-leaning Republican will dislike his film; both sides should look at facts and figures, not just opinions and hearsay. Rush Limbaugh vs. Al Franken if you will!

Maybe I should have picked a different film. If you are a liberal and want to believe in Michael Moore's film, more power to you! I have nothing against you. The point I want to make is that the Michael Moores of the world have the right to commit to film what they want to commit to film, and his detractors have the right to commit to any film that they want to commit to. Both groups have the right to say what they want to say.

Let's take another controversial subject: the JFK assassination. A casual filmgoer should not take as gospel what Oliver Stone has committed to film until he or she has looked at all the facts! After watching Oliver Stone's film, why not read Vincent Bugliosi's *Reclaiming History: The Assassination of President John F. Kennedy* and/or *Case Closed* by Gerald Posner. Both of those works take the view that Oswald killed Kennedy.

I'm not going to go into what I believe about that issue in this book either! I simply want to point out that someone who is truly open minded will look at all the facts before reaching a conclusion about what they believe. *JFK* was based on two books: *Crossfire, the Plot that Killed Kennedy* by Jim Marrs and *On the Trail of the Assassins* by Jim Garrison. It is my hope that someday, someone will make a movie based on Bugliosi's and Posner's books as well, just to give the debate a fair balance!

The conspiracy theorists have the right to film what they want, and people who believe that Oswald acted alone have the right to film what they want! The rest of us have an obligation to be intelligently informed rather than blissfully ignorant. The people who criticize *Wall-E* obviously don't know the statistics I'm talking about (blissfully ignorant), while the producers of this fine children's movie must have some idea of the facts (intelligently informed), and they want to use this information to help educate our young people to a problem which they are facing.

You have the right to dis Pixar if you want to, but I, and people like me, say kudos to the film makers at Pixar for trying to use their influence not just to entertain but to inform the young people of this country about a problem that can be corrected by their generation if they have the will to act on it! There! I've said my piece. Now let's talk about intelligent design vs. evolution . . . nah, just kidding; let's get back to discussing weight loss and the reason you bought this book in the first place: America's weight problem and what we can do about it, starting with you!

As I have noted, some people believe that by the year 2059, at the rate we are going, all Americans will be overweight! If you are reading this book and you are in any way overweight, apply the principles of this volume to your life, and we can begin to see the statistics for obesity go down in America, one person at a time!

If you see results after applying this program to your life, I want to know about it! Make sure you take some before and after photographs for proof that you have lost weight and send them to me along with your weight-loss story. The best stories will be included in my next book on weight loss.

As *Time* magazine points out, the first holiday established in this country was Thanksgiving—a holiday whose sole purpose was eating! It seems to be constantly on our minds; most business meetings are settled over lunch! Go to a party and what do you see? Hors d'oeuvres! A night of poker with the boys? Chips, dip, and beer! A woman's Tupperware party? Break out the cheesecake! Church social? Potluck supper!

Any type of gathering in this country seems to be centered on food! Americans, instead of eating to live, seem to be living to eat! So don't think it's going to be easy! If you want to get on a proper nutrition program, it will take some effort on your part, but don't get discouraged! You may cheat! I did; we all do. It's normal, but don't give up when you do! Just like riding a bike or a horse, when you fall off, get back on until you don't fall off.

Want more statistics to illustrate the trend? *Time* magazine again reports that in 1900 the average weight of a college age student was 133 lbs (male) and 122 lbs (female). By the year 2000 those weights had increased to 166 lbs (male) and 144 lbs (female). In 1985 there were only eight states where more than 10 percent of the adult population was obese; by 2006 there were no states in which the obesity level was that low, and in twenty-three states the number exceeded 25 percent.

For kids between two and five the number with a weight problem in 1971 was 5 percent but had gone up to about 14 percent by 2004. Those between age six and eleven in 1971 had a 4 percent obesity problem; by 2004 it had gone up to about 19 percent. Among those aged twelve to nineteen during that same period the number of obese kids went from 6.1 percent to 17.4 percent. These kids are seeing medical problems that they should not be seeing for many years to come: heart disease, liver disease, diabetes, gallstones, joint breakdown, and even brain damage. Many experts predict that today's youth could wind up with a shorter life expectancy than their parents.

One of the reasons for an increase in weight among our kids, of course, is that there is more to do around the house than there was in years gone by! This means less play and exercise time. In my day, all we had to keep us indoors was the vast wasteland that we called the television set. Today, there are personal computers, X-boxes, play stations, and any number of things to do around the house.

Our public schools are not helping the matter when they cut back on Phys Ed. (That's Physical Education, for those of us who remember.) In 1991, there were only about 42 percent of high school kids involved in any type of Phys Ed program, and today it's only about 25 percent. We need to get off our butts and get into shape! To put it bluntly!

2) MY STORY: HOW I LOST OVER 60 POUNDS WITH THE HELP OF A PERSONAL TRAINER

I had a rough time through the years keeping my weight down. I was obese. Let's not be polite—I was a fat slob! I tried for more than twenty years to lose weight! I tried every fad diet that came down the pike, only to lose a few pounds and then gain it back, with extra padding to spare. I tried them all: low-carb, low-fat, even an all-yogurt diet! Any diet that you can think of, all the popular diets of the day. I tried starvation diets, thinking that that would get rid of the fat! They all failed! As my instructor at the propta academy likes to say, I didn't fail the diet, the diet failed me! At my peak, I weighed 265 pounds!

Today I'm a slim 190 pounds and I eat what I want when I want to. I lost all my excess weight and I have succeeded in keeping it off. What's more, it's been easy. I wish that I'd known twenty years ago just how easy it would be. I had to learn how to lose the right weight the right way. If you know the secret, then you can do it! It is my intention to share with you the secret to losing weight and feeling great! Before I share that little secret with you, I want to tell you how I came to be obese and had to learn this little secret, which really isn't a secret.

When I was about five years old, my mother married my adoptive father, Joe Given. Without getting morbid or giving away the family secrets, I will say that Joe had a troubled first marriage and his first wife died under tragic circumstances. Joe blamed himself for her death and became an alcoholic. This was during my formative years, when other young boys were outside playing sports. I was inside, watching TV. I was the proverbial couch potato because, while my mother worked, someone had to stay home and watch Joe. Joe, of course, had lost his job by this time.

It is not my purpose to smear my stepfather's name in the writing of this chapter. I love my family and would not trade my upbringing for the world! I am not looking for sympathy or for anyone to feel sorry for me. I am very happy and I understand why things unfolded the way they did in my life! The reason that I'm sharing this with you is so that you will understand why I had gained the weight that I did.

Instead of going outside to play with the other kids, I was stuck at home, constantly eating and getting no exercise! My weight ballooned out. Joe would pass away while still in his forties, a victim of cirrhosis of the liver due to alcoholism (there were no liver transplants in those days). I was thirteen years old at the time. Of course, I was now free to go out and play with other kids, but I had become real depressed at being overweight.

I had very few friends and no reason to go outside, so I stayed home and watched *Star Trek* and *Brady Bunch* reruns until the news came on. Then my mother had control of the television and I would go to my room and listen to music: Kiss, Led Zeppelin, Aerosmith, Sweet, music that was considered heavy metal back then. By the time I was fourteen years old, I weighed 265 pounds—a lot of weight for a fourteen-year-old boy to be carrying around.

When I turned sixteen, I would become a born-again Christian. I found new friends by going to church, people who seemed to accept me, fat or not, and I enjoyed attending church services. Of course this book is not a theological treatise, so I'm not going to go into detail about that portion of my life; that's for another book. I simply want you to understand what motivated me during those years and helped me get through my childhood as I came up on adolescence.

When I turned eighteen, I realized that I was going to graduate high school soon, and I did not want to receive my diploma as a fat slob. I was also interested in a cute girl who was two years younger than me, so I went on my first diet! I lost thirty pounds by the time I graduated high school. I had finally succeeded at something!

What kind of diet helped me lose all that weight? It would be an all-yogurt diet! I ate nothing but two cups of yogurt a day for about six months. I don't remember how I decided on that diet, but that's what happened, and I lost the weight. Of course, this was not healthy, and shortly after graduating high school, I would regain the weight and then some!

After high school I went to Bible college. However, I would not finish, and I would then attend the University of Maine system as a speech/communications major. I then graduated from the New England School of Communications! I was now getting paid for what I loved doing: radio announcing!

Through the early years up until 1995 I worked at several radio stations in Maine: WRNE, WDHP, WREM, WOXO, and finally, the piece de resistance, my hometown radio station, WHOU in beautiful downtown Houlton, Maine. The station would go bankrupt within a year.

Most of the aforementioned stations would go bankrupt, and it would become increasingly difficult to get employment in radio. It was the mid-eighties and most stations were going automated. I had a killer demo tape, but why would a radio station hire a live DJ when a computer would do the job for free?

Again depression came upon me. I had spent all that money for three years of school, and I couldn't get employment in my chosen profession. Why complete my bachelor's degree if I would be working at Burger King after I got out? I could get a job at Burger King without an education, and that's precisely what I did! I worked at Burger King during the day and washed dishes at Ivey's Motor Lodge at night. This was not a high point of my vocational life, so I did what many twenty-somethings did for money, and I joined the National Guard.

Now, I told myself, I was really going to lose weight! I had my life all planned out. The intense workout that a soldier receives during army basic training would get me trimmed down. Then I would move back to Maine, get a decent radio job, and find Mrs. Right, get married, and live happily ever after; of course, this is real life, not a fairy tale!

It actually started to go that way! I lost a lot of weight and got down to 175 pounds, the slimmest I have ever been in my adult life! Within three months of leaving basic training, I would regain all the weight that I had lost! Why? Was I overeating? No! I ate normally and for a time I was still exercising every day; so what happened?

I had no idea why the blubber kept coming back. Every time I lost weight it seemed that it would come right back! Today I know why the weight would keep coming back, but we'll get to that in a few pages.

Many of you can relate to what I'm talking about as well as went through, and I know that you're itching to put the information to practical use, but I want you to get the complete picture of what I was going through, and besides, I have x amount of pages to fill up before I can call this a book, so patience please and we'll get there!

Army basic training was over! It was the mid-eighties and this was about the fourth time that I had lost and then regained weight. I did the all-yogurt diet, lost some weight, and gained it back. In college I went on the fad diet of the day, which was the Scarsdale Medical Diet, and there was also the intense workout called army basic training, which would get me to about five pounds of my ideal weight, which was 175 pounds, and even though I would eat normally, it would all come back every time. Was I doomed to a life of being overweight? Would my metabolism ever get right? For a long time I would just give up!

Depression set in once again! Not only was I discharged from the National Guard (honorably) for regaining all of my weight, but radio jobs were becoming even scarcer as it would become easier to automate than to hire a live DJ. I bounced around from one menial job to the next, usually fast food or security.

Let's move ahead to 1996; my friends had moved to Florida and had been trying to convince me to do the same thing. Finally, I would do just that! I left Maine on a Greyhound bus with fifty bucks in my pocket and a bag full of sandwiches that my mother had made me, peanut butter and jelly, MMM MMM good!

When I got to Florida, five of us were living in a two-bedroom apartment. I was running out of money and had to take the first job that I could get—Wendy's. I would work two jobs, the other being security, about sixty to eighty hours a week.

I tried the radio market in Florida but to no avail. That's when I met Mia (not her real name), who was a dancer and was dating a friend of mine at the time. She knew that I was trying to get radio work, and she would convince me to audition as a DJ at strip clubs, which I did!

Now, I know what some of you might be thinking: "Didn't you say that you had faith in God? What are you doing working in a place like that?" But again, I don't want to detract from the purpose of this book, which is my struggle with weight and how I overcame it, so I'll simply state that my decisions about God and my place of employment are another story for another book. I may not have always made the right decision in life, but that is what happened and I can't erase the past, only accept what happened, learn from it, and move on!

I was finally making money in the profession that I was trained in, and I was dating one of the prettiest girls I had ever met, Kasey. I wound up living with Kasey for two of the four years that we were together. Once again, I was happy, and once again, for those of you keeping score, my happiness would not last! Kasey and I would stop seeing each other and the money in that business would go downhill shortly after the turn of the century.

Sometimes I think that my name should be Charlie Brown, not Kevin Given. I mean good grief, can't I get decent steady employment? Of course, maybe the job decision was not the right one; even my non-religious friends told me that taking a job in that business would be a mistake. As I noted before, my decisions were not always right, but whose are? If you're perfect, please let me know so that I can find out how to become like you! But let's get to my last fad diet, the Atkins diet!

In the late nineties, some of the people that I worked with went on the Atkins diet and I saw them lose a little weight, so I thought I'd try it. At first I was amazed at how quickly I lost twenty pounds in like two weeks time! My eyesight even cleared up for a short time! I thought it was a miracle diet! I lost weight rapidly and didn't need glasses anymore! However, like all the other fad diets before it, the Atkins diet would fail, and as soon as I went off it I gained that weight back and then some!

Through the years, no matter how hard I tried, I couldn't keep the weight off! I would get down to about 230 pounds and then plateau. I was miserable and would once again regain the weight that I had lost, not to mention lose the 20/20 vision that I somehow regained and need new glasses again. So I gave up. I figured that there was no diet in the world that would work for me; I was destined to weigh about 260 pounds for the rest of my life! I simply accepted me for being me. "It is my metabolism," I lied to myself.

I soon moved to a different location, and as the fickle finger of fate would have it, my new location would re-route my path to work past a gym called Lifestyle Family Fitness Center in Largo, Florida. After passing that gym every day for several months, I finally got the urge to try and lose weight one more time. I was now in my forties, and I guess I was going through something of a mid-life crisis. I decided to stop in to talk to a personal trainer about my situation; boy am I glad that I did!

It was at "Lifestyle" that I met the personal trainer who would show me not only how to take off the weight but what I had been doing wrong all along. His name was Munier Neslanovic. Now I'm going to share with you the same secrets, which aren't really secrets, about weight loss that I have come to learn while training with Munier at Lifestyle Family Fitness Center. It was through this training that I learned how to apply these principles to my life and get into the shape that I had always wanted to be in.

Between 70 and 80 percent of your weight loss comes from proper nutrition, not exercise! So we can boil this down to two words: **Eat right.** The rest comes from exercise.

3) FAD DIETS BAD, NUTRITION PROGRAM GOOD!

First let's talk about low-carb diets. I went on a low-carb diet a few years ago, and I thought it was a miracle. I noticed a few of my co-workers losing weight and asked them how they were doing it. They told me, and I went on the same diet. At first, everything seemed to be going well. I lost weight and my vision even cleared up! That's right! I've had a vision problem since I was fourteen years old and my eyes were really bad, and when I went on this diet my eyesight became restored to 20/20 vision. I attribute this today to removing sugar totally from my diet; however, the good vision didn't last and my eyesight returned to what it was before the diet within a few months.

Once again I would plateau at about 230 pounds, and once again I got depressed to the point of regaining all my weight. Let's look at the problems associated with low-carb diets.

1) **Overeating fat is not healthy!** Common sense should tell you that you do not lose fat by overeating fat! Low-carb diets demand that you consume a lot of fat! Do you honestly think that the weight you have lost is fat when you are consuming three times the amount of fat that you should be? If you do believe that then I have some swamp land in the state of Florida for sale! The weight you are losing on this type of a diet is not fat, and you are doing your body serious damage! **STOP IT NOW!** Don't get me wrong. As we shall see, fat is essential in any nutrition program, but too much of anything is not good!

2) **High cholesterol:** Within a very few months, your cholesterol will rise, and each month you stay on that diet it will rise.

3) **Dehydration!** When you avoid carbohydrates, you will deplete the healthy glycogen stores in muscle and liver.

4) **Tiredness!** You won't feel like doing much of anything, including exercise, which you will need if you are to see results in a healthy fitness and nutrition program.

5) **Muscle atrophy:** Glycogen is the fuel of choice for muscle growth, and glycogen, as we have pointed out, depletes when you avoid carbohydrates.

6) **Basal metabolic rate decreases!** Metabolism happens in your muscle; a slower metabolism means fewer calories burned. You will actually have more fat on your body with a low-carb diet. As we pointed out, you do not lose fat by ingesting three times the amount of fat you should be eating!

7) **Muscles and skin sag:** This, of course, will lead to premature aging; how many of you can afford a plastic surgeon?

8) **Go off the diet; regain the weight!** I know of about twelve people who went on a low-carb diet, and only one of them managed to keep his weight down when he went off this diet! I consider him the exception that proves the rule! Everyone else, including me, gained it all back!

9 **Greater risks to your health!** A) Heart disease; B) strokes C) gallstones; D) kidney stones; E) arthritis; F) cancers (mostly of the digestive type).

10 **Lack of Fiber!** Animal products have no fiber. Only plant-based foods have fiber; this is one reason that the risk of digestive cancer increases (transit time is lengthened).

11 **Ketosis!** What is ketosis? This term is where the saying "Fat burns in the Flame of Carbohydrates" comes from! Without getting technical, ketosis is a type of metabolic acidosis. If fat is to burn efficiently and without excess toxic ketones, you must ingest enough carbohydrates. The body needs carbohydrates to function properly.

12 **Bad Breath!** You had better stock up on breath mints if you go on a low-carb diet! Altoids will become your best friend!

I'm not going to go into any more detail on these points, but if you want to learn more an excellent article on low-carb diets can be found on Greg Landry's web site: **www.greglandryfitness.com.** A proper nutrition program that will help you lose weight has to include the following: A) carbohydrates; B) protein; C) fat (yes, fat); D) vitamins; E) minerals; F) nutrients; G) water.

I got all that in army basic training! So I must have overeaten when I got out of boot camp, right? Wrong! So why did the weight come back after basic training? We ate the proper types of food, everything was steam cooked and properly prepared, and very little junk food was even offered to the soldiers during basic training. Well-balanced nutritional food was served every day and prepared properly. So what happened?

When I got out of basic, I continued to exercise and I ate fairly normally. You can imagine how shocked and confused I was when the weight started to come back! I was in my twenties, and I couldn't believe what was happening to me! Just as quickly as I lost the blubber it seemed to come back, and with a vengeance!

First month out of basic training—175lbs. Second month out of basic training—190lbs. Third month out of basic training—210lbs.

And so on until I got back up to 260 lbs.

What happened!? The simple answer is, the army works you to the bone and you lose weight the wrong way.

In short, don't work out on an empty stomach!

During army basic training they would get us up at about four or five a.m. and before eating anything we did a full day of exercise! I mean more exercise in one day than most people do in a month—a ten-mile run, sit-ups, pushups, chin-ups, squat thrusts, and more, for about three or four hours each day. Only after that workout did we eat breakfast. This was in 1986; I can only hope that they do not do this to soldiers today.

If anyone reading this is in any way connected with the military and has any influences whatsoever on their basic training practices, please get those soldiers to eat something before their P.T. (physical training)—a banana, a protein bar, anything. That way there will be something on their system that can be burned off and the body will not draw from their muscular system in the weight-loss process.

This way, the soldier will burn the right kind of weight and keep it off! The same thing goes for all of us! So many people who don't know what they're doing get up in the morning and hit the gym or start working out before they eat, only to do damage to their system!

We are not camels! We can't store food. The food that we consume is used when we consume it. So what happens when you exercise on an empty stomach? Your body will not have anything in the stomach to burn; it will draw from other sources, namely, your muscle! Think of your body as an automobile: You put fuel in it and drive! After you've gone about four hours you need to fuel up again, which leads me to my next point.

Do not eat three big meals per day!

As I said, and cannot stress enough, your body uses your food (fuel) when you consume it! It cannot be stored; therefore, if you overeat, then your body will use what you put into it, when you put it there! If you consume more than you need, then it will have no choice but to store the rest as FAT!

I don't know where the idea of three meals a day came from, but I do know that it is the wrong idea. Later on, I will show you an example of a basic nutritional outline, but for now, I simply wish to state that we need to consume small portions about every three hours. Once again, it's like putting fuel in a car; if you're using that fuel constantly, then it will be gone in three to four hours and you will need more. Do not eat big.

We've all seen ads for "UNICEF" and the "Christian Children's Fund" that show, tragically, starving kids in third-world countries, and those children have abnormally large bellies. Do you ever wonder why, since they are not eating right, their bellies are so big? It's because dieting and starvation are major factors in obesity. Why, when you go off of a fad diet, do you regain the weight lost and then some? It is because of a little enzyme called "lipoprotein lipase." When you go on a fad diet, or even worse, a crash starvation diet, your set point will go up, and your body reacts to try and protect you. Since you're not getting the aforementioned proteins, minerals, vitamins, carbohydrates, and nutrients it needs, the body will conserve energy by storing fat. The "lipoprotein lipase" will kick in in an attempt to return the reduced fat back to its original obese state. The body is desperately trying to compensate for not receiving the fuel it so urgently needs to keep it running right. It cannot perform the way it normally would when you take proper care of yourself. This is why fad diets are not good for your body.

When you go on a low-carb diet, your body will try to compensate for not getting the proper carbohydrates that it needs. When you go on a low-fat diet, or any other type of crazy diet and you deprive the body of fundamental substance, then your body will react in an effort to try and protect you the best way it can. That is why you will regain weight and then some when you go off whatever unhealthy diets you have put yourself on. Please stop risking your health with crazy diets and get on a proper nutrition plan today!

What of the vegetarian? Again, we're going to step on some toes. I do not wish to offend anyone who chooses a vegetarian diet for religious or social reasons. I have been taught to respect everyone's personal religious beliefs, and I try to live up to that respect. You can and do have the right to believe and follow whatever deity and religion that you worship; you also have the right not to believe in any particular faith, and I respect that right as well. Having said that, however, I must point out that human beings were meant to be omnivorous. Meat is an important part of the human diet.

Roughly eight to ten million of us profess to be vegetarians, and there are some studies that have been done to suggest that there are health benefits to being a vegan. These include lower rates of non-insulin-dependent diabetes mellitus and colon cancer. There are, however, many risks involved in skipping meat in our diets: 1) low iron; 2) slower metabolism; 3) low protein; 4) low levels of nitrogen; 5) amino acid deficiency.

A lack of these valuable resources for our bodies will lead to muscle deficiency, tiredness, and slower recovery from stress and illness. If you raise a child as a vegetarian that child will most likely be small for their age. Many vegetarians will consume poultry and fish, which will make up for many of the deficiencies that we've mentioned, but these people are not true Vegetarians, as the proud vegetarian will no doubt point out.

I respect your beliefs and your right to believe them, but if you are a true vegetarian, please find a way to compensate for your lack of eating meat with supplements. You need protein and other healthy resources that meat gives us.

4) A BEGINNERS GUIDE TO A WEEKLY NUTRITION PROGRAM

Now we're going to talk about nutrition! I said near the beginning of this book that I was glad McDonalds won a case where they were sued for causing two girls to gain weight, and I stand by that. When it comes to our public schools, I definitely have a different viewpoint. Fatty foods should not be offered to our kids at school! If they are offered nothing but healthy foods then they can't eat garbage.

If you pack your kid's lunch then you should know how to feed your own kids. Now, if your kids are going to sneak off to McDonalds during lunch, well, until you find out, then there's not much you can do about it, except maybe not let them have the money that they need to take off for a junk-food-filled afternoon!

Some schools are taking the initiative and not offering soda and snack machines on their premises, which is a good thing! Fruits for dessert instead of candy bars; grilled chicken instead of fried chicken, vegetables instead of potato chips. These are steps we can all take, not just the schools, to see our kids get healthy and stay healthy.

One of the problems in American society, though, is denial. Do you admit that your child is overweight? Most likely, you do not, and you are in the majority. The same *Time* magazine article that we looked at earlier shows that only 36 percent of parents who had obese children between the ages of two and seventeen identified those children as being overweight. It is speculated that some of the reasons for this state of denial are manifold. **1) Their kids no longer have baby fat.** This makes their present weight look acceptable, even when it's not! **2) Not wanting to hurt our own children's feelings.** We are sensitive to the way our kids perceive themselves and want them to feel good about themselves, so we deny those love handles too; **3) Since obesity is becoming the norm, a slightly overweight child is perceived as not being that bad!** My kid is slimmer than your kid! But that, of course, does not make the child healthy.

Because of these stages of denial, many doctors find it hard to discuss a child's weight problem with the parents, even when it's obvious, plainly obvious, that the child has one. Many parents will change the subject or flat out tell their physician that little Johnny or Mary does not have a weight problem that they will eventually grow out of it! Some parents can get downright hostile when the doctor is only trying to help. "How dare he" they will think.

Experts believe that these stages of denial make it difficult for the physicians to give simple advice that the whole family should heed, not just the kids: **1) Eat five or more servings of fruits and vegetables daily; 2) get a minimum of one hour of physical activity per day; 3) spend fewer than two hours a day in front of any screen**

Our behaviors are imitated by our kids. If they see us doing something bad, or good, for ourselves, then they will probably do the same or similar activities. One good example is smoking. If we smoke, it's most likely that our kids will smoke, and vice versa. So we have to teach our kids by example.

The time has to be now, because, according to the Department of Health and Human Services (HHS), seven out of ten overweight kids will become overweight adults and will not grow out of it! So it stands to reason that if we gain weight, our kids will gain weight, based on the argument that we just presented. Let's take a look at a healthy week of eating right. Here is an example of a weekly nutrition program that can work:

> <u>Monday Breakfast</u> (Do not skip the most important meal of the day!): two eggs, any style, 1/2 avocado, 1/2 cup of potatoes, diced. <u>Snack</u> (about three hours after breakfast): 3/4 cup of plain nonfat yogurt with 3/4 mixed dried fruits. **<u>Lunch</u>** (three hours after the snack): three ounces of tuna salad on a bed of lettuce; this doesn't require dressing. **<u>Snack</u>** (three hours after lunch): soy butter, half a slice of bread, and apricot spread. **<u>Dinner</u>** (three hours after the snack): four ounces of firm tofu diced and cubed; 1/2 cup of mushrooms, green peppers, carrots, broccoli; olive oil; 1/2 teaspoon of soy sauce diluted with vinegar; and 1/2 cup of rice. **<u>Snack</u>** (three hours after dinner): one cup of nonfat yogurt sweetened with one cup of fresh strawberries.

Make sure that you eat every three hours; going hungry will not help you lose weight! You must maintain a healthy diet! This will be 70 to 80 percent of your weight-loss success.

Tuesday Breakfast: two egg whites, one cup of oatmeal and Lactaid milk. **Snack:** 3/4 cup of plain non-fat yogurt with 3/4 cup of blueberries. **Lunch:** four ounces of flat-iron steak, steamed vegetables, 1/2 of a plain baked potato. **Snack:** 1/2 cup of chicken salad, 1/2 grapefruit. **Dinner:** four egg whites, diced vegetables (bell peppers, mushrooms, carrots) all mixed while cooked. **Snack:** one wedge of pumpkin pie with non-dairy whipped cream.

Yes, you can have things like pumpkin pie; if prepared properly, of course. Does this diet look tasty so far? Think you can handle it? Without cheating? Well don't be discouraged if you do find yourself failing, especially in the beginning. Everyone has cheated, but once again, just like riding a horse or a bike, don't give up but get back on! And keep reading, because we'll get into having a cheat day every once in a while. You will get to eat some foods that you like and still maintain optimum weight loss! You may have cravings when you first start a nutrition program, but they will eventually disappear as you begin to eat healthy!

Wednesday Breakfast: two eggs scrambled with two ounces of ground chicken, 1/2 cup of potatoes, diced. **Snack:** sliced apple with soy (peanut) butter. **Lunch:** Four ounces of chicken stir-fried with vegetables and olive oil; 1/2 teaspoon of teriyaki sauce. **Snack:** soy butter; 1/2 sliced banana; one slice bread. **Dinner:** three ounces of any fish, 1/2 baked potato, steamed vegetables (unlimited). **Snack:** 3/4 cup of plain nonfat yogurt mixed with one cup strawberries.

Some people ask me about protein bars. If you are in a pinch and have a job where you don't have much time on break, then you could substitute a protein bar for a snack, but generally I would say to avoid them because their fat content is generally higher than the snacks in our program. The same, of course, goes for protein shakes. If you have absolutely no choice in the matter, use them, but, when possible, avoid them. They are OK if you need to get something and you know you won't have time to prepare a snack. When you have a day off though, stick with the snacks in our program.

Thursday Breakfast: one cup of nonfat yogurt, one pack of sweetener, and 1/2 cup of honeydew melon. **Snack:** one wedge of sugar-free apple pie. **Lunch:** shrimp salad (sliced small) with fat-free mayonnaise on a bed of lettuce. **Snack:** one cup of nonfat yogurt sweetened with one cup of raspberries. **Dinner:** three ounces of chicken dipped in egg whites and breaded and slightly baked with steamed vegetables. **Snack:** 3/4 cup of plain nonfat yogurt with 3/4 ounce of granola.

This diet so far is very rich in all of the substances your body needs for its daily intake. You will get a healthy dose of protein, carbohydrates, and fat, vitamins, minerals and nutrients. After two weeks on this diet, you should see a significant drop in excess weight. If, for some reason, you do not, consult with a nutritionist. Of course, if the reasons that you do not see weight loss are due to your not staying on the nutrition program, then you cannot blame the program for your lack of weight loss. Look in a mirror, and that is who you will have to blame! Let's stay on program!

Friday Breakfast: one cup of nonfat yogurt, one packet of sweetener, 1/2 cup of cantaloupe. **Snack:** 3/4 cup of yogurt mixed with 3/4 cup of mixed nuts and dried fruits. **Lunch:** Three ounces of any fish (not fried), 1/2 cup of wild rice, and 1/2 avocado. **Snack:** one cup of nonfat yogurt with one cup of fresh strawberries. **Dinner:** three ounces of chicken salad on a medium bed of lettuce; does not require dressing. **Snack:** soy butter, half slice of bread, and apricot spread.

The weekend is here! We're almost through the first week; hang tough, in one week those cravings for good-tasting but fattening food will be gone! Let's talk about a cheat day! Now, when I say you can have a cheat day, I don't mean to overindulge! Don't say, "I've got a cheat day so I can eat as much as I want!" Eat a little bit of what you like! If you're into pizza, then have a slice, maybe two, at dinner time. Don't eat an entire large pizza by yourself! A cheat day can actually help you lose weight as it will shock the system. You will be changing your eating habits on a cheat day!

Saturday Breakfast: two eggs, any style, 1/2 avocado, 1/2 cup of potatoes, diced. **Snack:** 3/4 cup of plain nonfat yogurt with 3/4 cup of blueberries. **Lunch:** four ounces of chicken stir-fried with vegetables and olive oil, 1/2 teaspoon of teriyaki sauce diluted with vinegar. **Snack:** one wedge of pumpkin pie with non-dairy whipped cream. **Dinner:** three ounces of chicken dipped in egg whites and breaded and slightly baked with steamed vegetables. **Snack:** 3/4 cup of plain nonfat yogurt mixed with one cup strawberries.

We'll take Sunday and make it a cheat day! Now you do not have to make Sunday your cheat day. This nutrition plan is simply a guide; you do not have to follow it exactly. If you do not like yogurt, substitute for it with simple fruits and/or fruit salad (no syrup). A cup of grapes mixed with almonds could be one of your snacks; anything that is healthy, nutritious, and nonfattening. If you are really hungry, make a huge plate of steamed vegetables with grilled chicken or fish. Don't let yourself go hungry; you will only do damage.

Sunday The final day, or first day, depending on how you look at it, we'll call a cheat day. **Breakfast:** two egg whites, one cup of oatmeal, and Lactaid milk. **Snack:** 3/4 cup of yogurt mixed with 3/4 cup of mixed nuts and dried fruits. **Lunch:** three ounces of tuna salad on a bed of lettuce; this doesn't require dressing. **Snack:** soy butter, 1/2 sliced banana, 1 slice bread. **Dinner:** whatever you want, within reason! If you want fast food, eat one burger, not three. Pizza, one or two slices, not an entire large. This is your time to eat your favorite food, but be careful; you do not want to regain what you lost. **Snack:** soy butter, 1/2 sliced banana, one slice bread.

Now let's talk about supplements. If you are going to enter a serious workout program, you will want to take at least two multivitamins per day; if you are working out to a great degree, make it three. You may want to take some other form of protein, like a shake or a snack, along with amino acids and other forms of supplements. Consult a trainer before doing so. I cannot give more advice here, since I don't know your workout or your goals. We'll talk more about it later.

Using the same *Time* magazine article that we discussed at the beginning of the book, let's look at how nutrition has changed for public school students.

A typical 1950s school lunch:

Food:

Calories:
   Bread and butter 142
   Whole milk 150
   Peas and corn 60
   Mashed potatoes & pot roast 584
   Total calories (39 percent recommended daily intake) 936

Let's look at a typical modern school lunch:

Food:

Calories:
   Chocolate chip cookie 300
   Peaches 80
   Mexican rice 190
   Orange juice 95
   Refried beans 90
   Salsa & nachos 418
   Total calories (49 percent recommended daily intake) 1,173

The following chart is how today's lunch should be:

Food:

Calories:
   Strawberries 25
   Carrots and dip 136
   Low-fat milk 100
   Vegetable soup 100
   Turkey wrap & grapes 237
   Total calories (27 percent recommended daily intake) 648

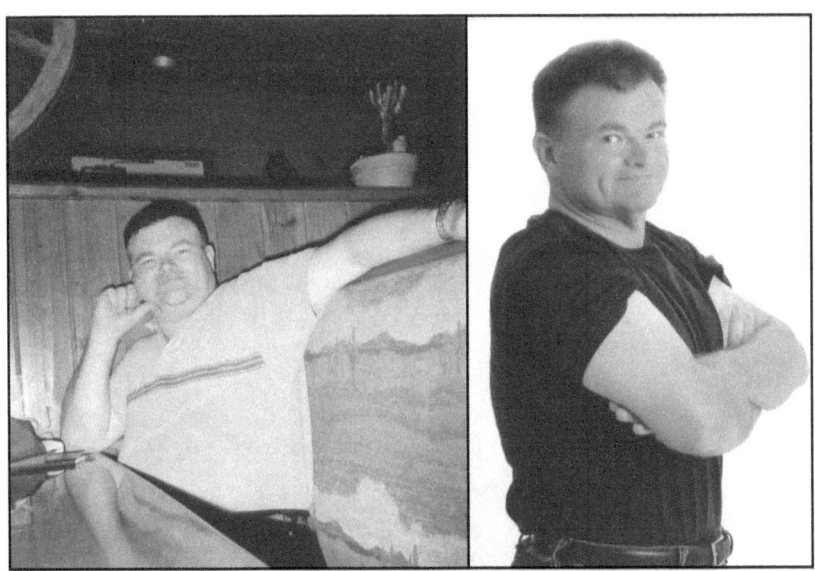

Before hiring a personal trainer; after hiring a personal trainer

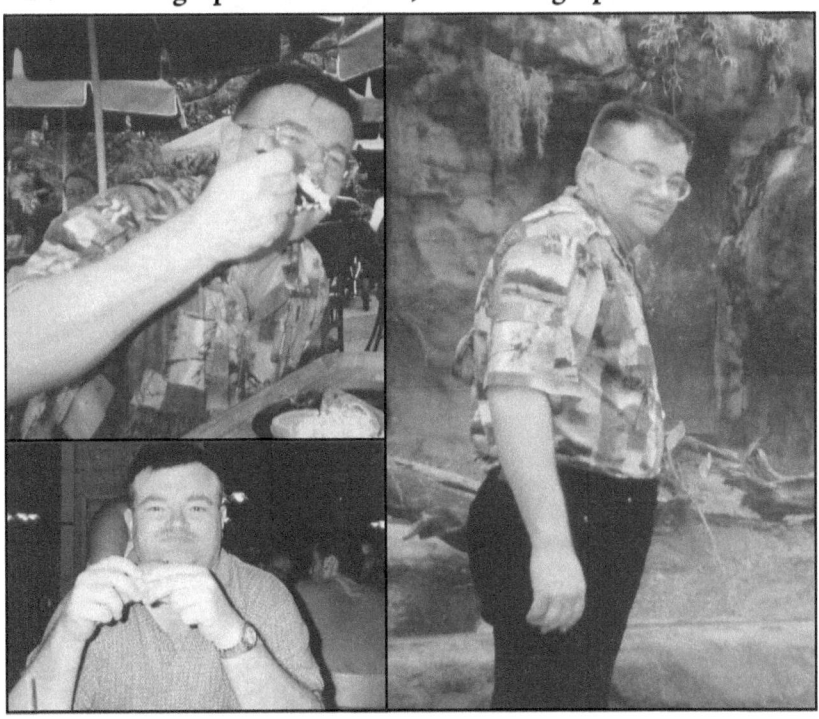

One thing's for sure, I knew how to eat! Hello Newman!

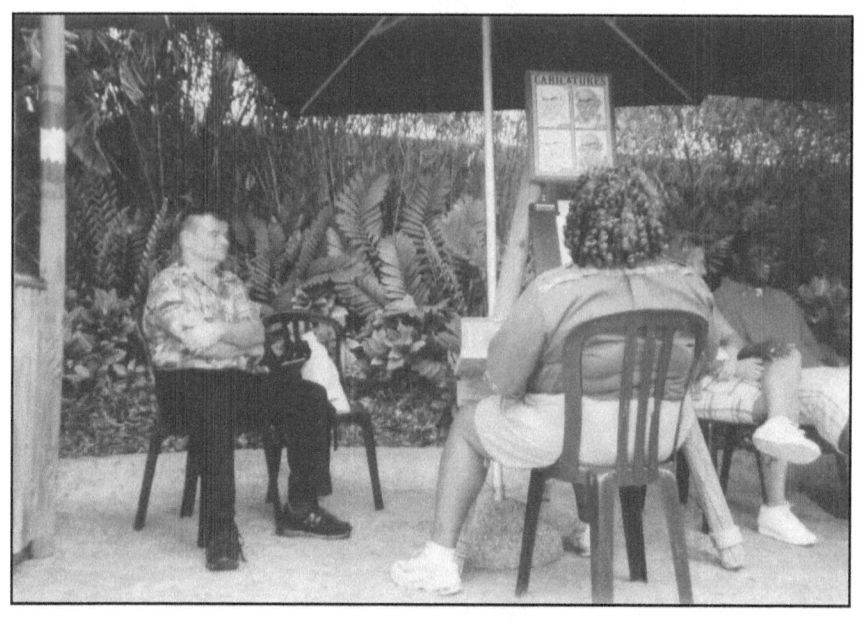

Getting my caricature drawn on my honeymoon at Busch Gardens, Florida

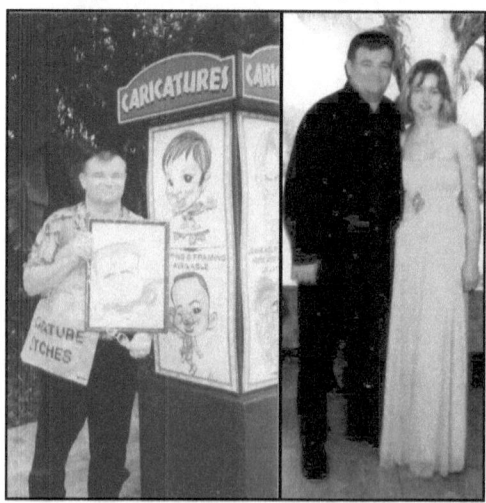

I'm a Superhero! With my beautiful wife, Beata!

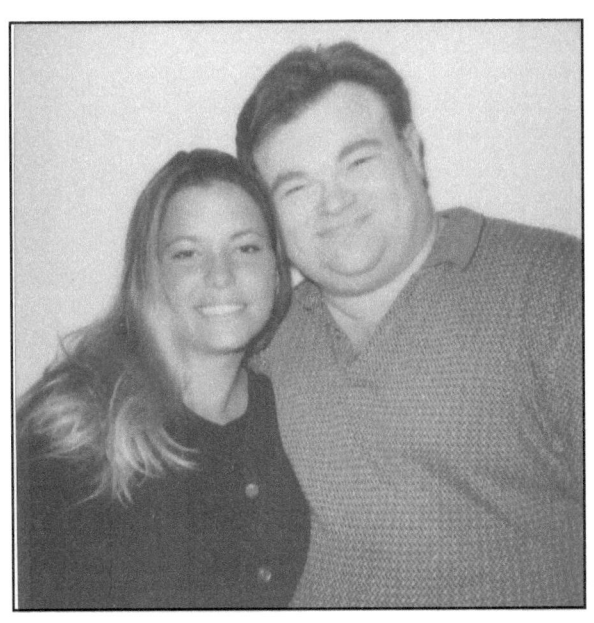

Kasey, an ex-girlfriend and I, around 2005!
This was me at my heaviest: 265 pounds!

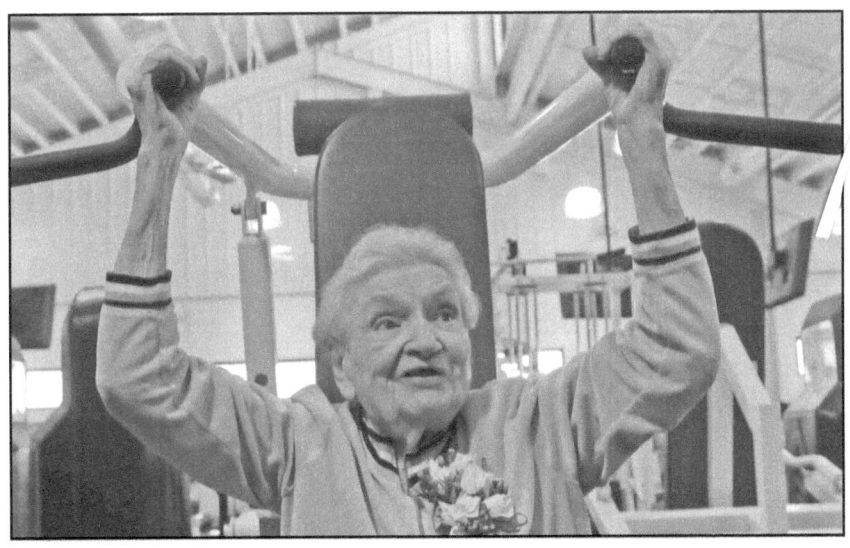

Ida Wasserman, the miracle lady that started
working out at the age of 100.

5) A BEGINNERS GUIDE TO A WEEKLY WORK-OUT PROGRAM

Now that we've looked at nutrition, I want to give you a basic chapter on weight resistance training. But I must caution you not to enter any type of a fitness program unless you know what you are doing. You will only cause damage to your system. At least consult a physician before exercising.

1) Warm up! Before you do any type of exercise it is important that you warm up first. This will prevent damage to ligaments and tendons and prevent injury. Your warm-up will consist of stretching, walking or light treadmill, and lifting light weights. **A) Stretching.** When you stretch the limbs, your muscles should be relaxed. You must also be careful not to overdo the stretch or you can do serious damage to ligaments and tendons. Make sure you stretch your arms, shoulders, and elbow area as well as your legs, hamstrings, and thighs. This will make for a body that is prepared for resistance weight training. If you do not stretch your limbs, you will do serious damage to your body. **B) Walking or treadmill.** This will help loosen all the muscles, especially in the legs. Do ten-minute walks or a five-minute treadmill run prior to weight training. **C) Light weight lifting.** Again, this will help loosen your arm muscles and prevent soreness to the limbs. After this workout, you are ready to begin!

2) Strength training: This is also called weight training or resistance training. If you are trying to lose a lot of weight then it is important to do your weight training before your cardiovascular training (excluding the five-minute warm up, which we do before the strength training). This will help you burn fat! If you do not do strength training before aerobics or cardiovascular (cardio) training, then you will burn more muscle than you want to!

When you work out, your body will draw from all its resources! If you do strength training before the cardio, you will use the muscles and only burn 10 percent muscle during your cardio workout. If, however, you do not do strength training before your cardio training, you will not use your muscles before the workout and you will burn 30 percent muscle during this phase of the workout and 70 percent fat! It would obviously benefit you to burn more fat during the cardio or aerobic workout, especially if you have a lot of fat to burn. So do your strength training before your cardio training, and you will be all the better for it!

Now let's take a look at a sample schedule for a week of intense training with the goal of reducing weight. Then we will discuss the stretches and exercises in each example.

First we'll start with an exercise week for the female. As women and men have different metabolisms, their workouts will be slightly different. **Resistance training:** This will help you build muscles, giving curve and shape to your form. It will not create huge bulky arms, which most woman fear, and it will work to avoid what are called bat wings, or flabby arms. Each workout will begin with a warm-up, five minutes on the treadmill. Also stretch the limbs, to help prevent soreness. Each day will work a different body part: Monday, upper body; Tuesday, lower body; Wednesday, a rest day; Thursday, upper body; Friday, lower body; and Saturday, upper body; Sunday will be another rest day.

Overhead extensions: You will lie on your back on a bench and hold a barbell extended out in front of you. Slowly and in a controlled manner you will lower the bar past your forehead, keeping the elbows close to your head. Once you have lowered it as far as you can go you will bring it back to the starting position. **Lying triceps extensions:** You will lie on your back on a bench and hold a barbell extended out in front of you. Slowly and in a controlled manner, you will lower the bar right past the forehead, keeping the elbows close to your head. Once you have lowered it as far as you can, you will bring it back to the starting position, contract the triceps, and repeat. **Bench dips:** You will place your palms on the bench behind you. Extend your feet out in front of you, toes up, and bend your knees. Slowly and in a controlled manner, keeping your elbows stationary and close to your body, lower your body down as far as you can. Be sure to keep your body close to the bench. Using the triceps, rise back and contract your triceps, and repeat the movement. To work the front of your arms (biceps), try the following. **Barbell curls:** Hold the barbell in front of you with your palms facing outward. In a slow and controlled manner, curl the bar up toward your chest area; squeeze your biceps, and release. Repeat. **Alternate dumbbell curls:** Hold a dumbbell in each hand with your palms facing your body. In a controlled manner, curl each one up individually and rotate the wrist so your palm is facing your shoulder when the curl is in the contracted position. Slowly release and repeat. **Squats:** Squats work the entire leg and "glute" muscle. If you skip the squats, you are doing yourself a great disservice. To begin, choose a weight you are comfortable with. Stand with your feet shoulder-width apart. Keep your back straight and lower yourself until your knees are at a ninety-degree angle. Make sure you contract your "glutes" at the top of the movement and drive the power through your heels. Perform three sets with light to moderate weight in the fifteen-to-twenty-repetition range with one-minute rest intervals. Don't use excessively heavy poundage if you carry most of your weight in your hips, thighs, and buttocks. **Stiff-legged dead lifts**: The stiff-legged dead lifts also help to work the "glutes" as well as the hamstrings. This is often a neglected exercise. Form is important. Keep your focus on your hamstrings and "glutes" and not the back. To begin, choose a weight that you are comfortable with. Stand with your feet shoulder-width apart and hold the weight in front of you. While keeping your lower back tight, slowly drop your hips behind you and allow the weight to fall toward your feet. As you rise, squeeze and contract your hamstrings and "glutes." Perform three sets of stiff-legged dead lifts with light to moderate weight in the fifteen-to-twenty-repetition range with one-minute rest intervals. **Lunges:** Lunges work the entire leg and "glute" area. You can choose to do this with or without weights. To begin, stand normally. Lunge one foot forward until the knee is at a ninety-degree angle, and then resume standing position. Do the same movement for the other legs. Perform three sets of lunges with light to moderate weight in the fifteen-to-twenty-repetition range with one-minute rest intervals.

Resistance training will build firm and toned "glutes," but in order to remove the fat, cardiovascular exercise is needed. Any aerobic exercise is good for burning calories and burning fat, but choosing the ones that target the legs and "glutes" are even better. Power walking, jogging, sprinting, in-line skating, and the elliptical are the best for leaning up the lower body and "glutes." Perform these at least three times a week for twenty minutes and progress each week from there. The stepper and treadmill are great for glutes and buttocks, but if you are not after increased size, avoid them each day. You will work out for forty-five minutes with fifteen minutes for warm up and cool down and do three sets of ten reps for each exercise for that day.

Now let's set up a workout regimen for the men: As with the female Men should work out for forty-five minutes with fifteen minutes for warm up and cool down, doing three sets of ten reps each. Monday will be upper body, Tuesday will be lower body, and Wednesday will be a rest day! Thursday will be for upper body, Friday will be for lower body, and Saturday will be for upper body, with Sunday being another rest day. The exercises for the male will be similar to those for women; however, we will concentrate on building muscle rather than shaping curves. **Front lateral raise:** Grasp dumbbells in front of thighs. Bend over at hips slightly with knees bent. With elbow slightly bent, raise upper arms to sides, slightly to the front, until shoulder height. Maintain elbow height above or equal to wrists.

Dumbbell shrugs: Stand holding dumbbells to sides and then elevate the shoulders as high as possible; lower and repeat. **Barbell shrugs:** Stand holding barbell with an overhand or mixed-grip shoulder width or slightly wider. Elevate the shoulders as high as possible. Lower and repeat. **Upright rows:** Grasp bar with shoulder width or slightly narrower overhand grip. Pull the bar up to the neck with elbows leading. Allow wrists to flex as bar rises. Lower and repeat. **Preacher curls:** Using a preacher curl bench and an EZ curl bar, make sure the seat is adjusted to the right height. When you sit, the seat should not be so low that the shoulders are elevated nor so high that you're hunched over the pad. Grasp the bar using a shoulder-width grip. Curl the bar upward in an arc. As you begin, be careful not to swing or rock to get it moving. The goal is to make the exercise hard on the biceps. Curl the bar towards your chin, but keep in mind that the resistance is greater at the beginning of the rep. Go down SLOWLY and work the muscle on the way down as well. This can also be done with two dumbbells or one arm at a time. **Concentration curls:** Begin seated on a bench or chair. Hold a dumbbell with an underhand grip, resting that elbow on the inner side of your thigh. Lower the weight back down until your arm is straight but the elbow is not locked. **Barbell curls:** With your hands shoulder-width apart, grip a barbell with an underhand grip. Stand straight up with your shoulders squared and with your feet shoulder-width apart. Let the bar hang down at arm's length in front of you, with your arms, shoulders, and hands in a straight line. WITHOUT leaning back or swinging the weight, curl the bar up toward your chest in an arc. Keep your elbows in the same place and close to your sides. Bring the weight up as high as you can and squeeze your biceps at the top. Lower the weight slowly, resisting all the way down until your arms are nearly straight. **Dumbbell curls:** To start, have a seat on the incline bench with both arms hanging down the sides holding the dumbbells. Make sure that your arms are perpendicular to the floor and your palms are facing each other. Starting with one arm, proceed to curl the dumbbell up, twisting at the wrist so that your palm is facing up. Curl the dumbbell while keeping the upper arm perpendicular to the floor. Pause for one second and then bring the weight down. Other exercises will include **Chest:** bench press, chest press machine, pushups, pec-deck machine; **Back:** seated row machine, back extensions, lat pull downs; **Shoulders:** overhead press, lateral raise, front raise; **Biceps:** bicep curls, hammer curls, concentration curls; **Triceps:** triceps extensions, dips, kickbacks; **Lower body:** squats, lunges, leg press machines, dead lifts, calf raises; **Abdominals crunches:** reverse crunches, oblique twists, pelvic tilts. I cannot stress enough for beginners, especially if you are over forty, not to go into a workout program blindly. Do not simply take the exercises that I have just listed and run to a gym and sign up. Consult a trainer and/or a physician to see what's right for you! We'll talk more on that in our next chapter. But right now I want to point out that these workouts must be done correctly or they will be ineffectual!

The amount of the weight is unimportant when your goal is to tone the body. If you do not experience full range of motion with a sticking point, then you are not exercising the muscle. Some of you might be asking what is full range of motion. **Full range of motion** is how we measure the effectiveness of the exercise. If the exercise is not executed properly, then you will not be working the muscle. Without going into detail, you must recruit all muscle fibers to perform an effective weight training exercise. If the exercise is not performed correctly, then you have done the muscle no good whatsoever. You will be more effective with five or ten pounds performing the exercise correctly then you would be with thirty or forty pounds yet performing the exercise incorrectly. If you cannot do the exercise with whatever weight you are using then lower the weight! **Sticking Point:** The sticking point is simply the point where it is hardest to do the exercise. It's at the sticking point that you are actually working the muscle. If you miss the sticking point, you will not be working the muscle at all! The descriptions of these and more exercises can be found on the web at:

http://www.womenfitness.net

http://en.wikipedia.org/wiki/Strength_training

http://www.weight-lifting-workout-routines.com

http://www.explosivelyfit.com

http://female.bodybuildbid.com

http://exercise.about.com

http://www.seriousstrengthtraining

6) THE IMPORTANCE OF A CERTIFIED PERSONAL TRAINER

It is important that you go into any fitness program with a proper understanding of what you are doing to your body. If you want to lose weight and keep it off, or if you're just trying to get into good physical shape, a fitness program is important to consider. If you go about it blindly then you will do more damage than good to yourself. I highly recommend that you hire a certified personal trainer to assist you with your goals, no matter what they may be! A certified personal trainer knows how to assess the ways you need to achieve your goals. As I said at the beginning of this book, I tried for years to lose weight, going into different programs either blindly or armed with only half the knowledge that I needed to accomplish my goals. As a result I did more damage than good to my body.

Today I have lost the weight and kept it off! Before I might have lost a couple of pounds only to see them come back and then some! Fad diets don't work; a proper nutrition program does. Grabbing weights without knowing how to properly execute the exercise that goes with them is dangerous and will do more harm than good. Lifting the weight properly will help develop those muscles and get them into shape.

I have given you many good guidelines in this book to help you achieve your goals, but in the end, I don't know you! Unless I get to know you I cannot develop a plan for you personally, I don't know your age, your sex, your weight, your height, your metabolism. I have no idea how to develop a successful program for you. In short, hire a personal trainer. You'll be glad that you did!

At the end of this chapter I will give you contact information for me and other personal trainers who can help you in ways that you cannot imagine. After all, you've probably tried everything you can on your own and failed; can it hurt to call a personal trainer? As I have stated on the back of this book, what do you have to lose? Except more weight! Before we look at the benefits of hiring a personal trainer, I want to look at what can go wrong if you enter a physical fitness program blindly. The older you get, the more damage that can be done if you haphazardly try to lose weight or get into shape without knowing how! If you are over forty, don't even think of entering a gym on your own! And I mean that!

1) Incorrect posture: Many people don't even know if they are using the correct posture when they exercise. A certified personal trainer who knows what they are doing will guide you and show you the proper stance you need to take. Working out with incorrect posture will lead to a deformed or disfigured body! Where do you think hunchbacks come from? **2) Working out too long!** Another big mistake almost all amateurs, including myself, make is to stay in the gym too long! This will cause more damage than good! I thought that the more time that I spent in the gym, the more fat I would burn; this is so totally wrong! You will not help yourself; once you have burned off what fat you can for the day, you will burn no more! How long is right for you? A trainer who knows what he or she is doing will be able to tell you. **3) The wrong amount of cardio training!** For some people, unlike myself, their problem isn't trying to lose weight; it's trying to gain weight! They have a high-speed metabolism and will skip cardio training sometimes altogether. These people will gain the wrong kind of weight and get fat with no or not enough cardio training. On the other hand, people like me who try to burn off fat, thinking that they have to spend two or three hours with a cardio workout, will lose the wrong kind of weight and see what weight they lose come right back on their body. Find out what's right for your metabolism and do it the right way! **Breathing right:** Breathe out as you lift the weight and breathe in as you lower the weight. Why is this important? Improper breathing can do serious damage, especially to the heart. I know of one young lady whose father was a body builder who died in his early forties due to little tears in his heart; otherwise he was perfectly healthy! It was speculated that his breathing technique was improper! Some medical conditions that can develop due to improper training may include **blood pressure elevation, retinal hemorrhages** (causing vision damage), **aneurysms,** and **rhabdomyolysis** (pain and swelling of the muscle

A personal trainer is there to monitor your progress and make sure that you are careful enough to prevent these problems and injuries. Now, this does not mean that you won't necessarily get hurt—even with a personal trainer you may still get injured—but having a trainer (I must stress, a certified trainer) will definitely reduce the risks of injuries developed during training.

Of course, preventing injuries is not the only reason to hire a personal trainer. **Motivation** is another key to weight loss. If you have an appointment with a personal trainer at a gym, you are more likely to show up and work out! Think of it. If you go on your own, how many times do you miss a workout? A trainer can be a lot like a drill instructor, getting you to go the extra mile! You show up because you're expected to. You will not miss that workout also because you've paid to be there. If you are not there then that is money out of your pocket.

If the military sent a soldier to basic training with only an army manual and no guidance, that soldier wouldn't learn much! How many soldiers would get up at four or five a.m. without the drill sergeants going through the hall with a stick and a garbage can banging as loudly as he or she can? Who would be motivated to do pushups if the drill sergeant didn't yell, "Drop and give me twenty"? Just as the soldier is guided to his peak performance during army basic training, so an individual seeking to get into better shape will be guided by the personal trainer into reaching his/her goal! Call one today! It's your health and there's no time like the present. It's your body, it's your life, and it's time to take charge and enjoy it for a change! **Setting up realistic goals:** The physical fitness trainer will calculate how much you need to lose (or gain) and show you how to achieve your goals. They will calculate body fat, take you on a week-by-week guide to optimal wellness, and do everything in their power to see that you will reach the goals that you set forth, together! It's easier to get things done when there is more than one person involved! You know that other old saying "It takes two to tango"? Two people can always reach a goal easier than one.

It's also much easier to reach a goal if you focus on the outcome of a project on a week-by-week basis. Is it worth the investment? Tell me when you look in the mirror and like what you see as opposed to avoiding mirrors! Tell me when you start to spend more time at the beach instead of away from it and you get more stares from the opposite sex! I think that you'll agree, in the end, that it was well worth the money spent to hire that personal trainer!

Getting to know more about your body: Someone who has studied the human metabolism can guide you to a more physically fit you! If you are over thirty, then there are things happening inside of you that can affect the outcome of your workout. Each decade after that sees greater risk for harm in an uncontrolled workout environment. For instance, in physically inactive people there is a loss of about 3–5 percent muscle mass per decade and a parallel decline in strength. If you have been largely inactive into your thirties, you have lost a lot of muscle use that you may not even notice!

You know the old saying "Use it or lose it"? That is so true in regards to the human body! People who go on liquid diets tend to lose their teeth because they are not using them! Likewise, muscles that lie dormant will lose strength. If you are really inactive you could develop sarcopenia or osteoporosis. Keeping active helps to prevent, or at least delay, these types of muscle atrophy. Those of us who were smart started working out before we hit thirty; unfortunately, I was not one of the smart ones!

There are a lot of reasons why you should at least consult an expert before engaging in a physical fitness program, especially if you are over thirty. I am not going to touch on all of them in this book; however, there is one more I would like to mention: **stress-related injury.** So many people do not realize that stress plays an important role in hindering our optimal goals in a workout session. When we are stressed, the level of oxygen that reaches our blood is changed; therefore the muscle does not reach the optimal workout that it could achieve, and of course, if we are concentrating on whatever it is that is causing stress, then we won't be concentrating 100 percent on our workout session.

We should not be stressed out at the time of a workout or we will not achieve the goal we have set for that workout. How can we reduce stress prior to a workout? The simplest way is to stop concentrating on whatever is causing the stress and put our minds on other things. If we have difficulty doing that, then we should think nutritionally!

Cortisol production is very important to the athlete, and stress will change the amount of cortisol produced in the trainee. It has been shown that vitamin C can reduce stress during a workout. Drinking a sports drink high in carbohydrates during a workout will help. This will produce insulin release, which can offset the production of cortisol. This will control the fluctuations brought on by weight resistance training.

To summarize, the benefits of having a personal trainer include:

1) Help to prevent injuries.

2) Knowledge of what works for you in nutrition.

3) Knowledge of what works for you in weight training.

4) Motivation.

5) Setting up realistic goals.

6) Getting to know more about your body.

It's your body. Do you want to get into better shape? If you need a personal trainer and are living in the greater Los Angeles area, I am currently taking applications.

Contact information:

Kevin Given

My personal cell phones: 310-536-6052;

My web site: http://trainerkevingiven.tripod.com/

My e-mail address: legendsofrock2003@yahoo.com

If I have reached my goal in clientele, you can contact the professionals at the Private Trainers Association at propta.com.

7) IT'S NEVER TOO LATE TOO START

"It won't do me any good to work out. I'm too old!" I am so tired of hearing people say that they are too old to work out or to begin a fitness program because it won't do them any good at their age! A fitness program will benefit you at any age! How old is too old anyway? Thirty, forty, fifty, sixty, seventy, eighty? Ninety? Can a ninety-year-old really benefit from joining a fitness program? How about one hundred? If by some miracle you live to be one hundred years old and have been inactive, can you really begin a fitness program and see results? I say yes!

Some of you reading this book are probably laughing out loud right now! Is he crazy? People at that age can't work out; they'll have heart attacks, won't they? He can't really know anybody that's one hundred years old and started working out! That's crazy; it's impossible! Tell that to Ida Wasserman. You don't know Ida Wasserman? Well let me tell you about this incredible lady!

Ida is over one hundred years old. A few years ago, Ida was living in New York and had been diagnosed with severe osteoporosis. She couldn't move without the aid of a walker. Ida was all hunched over and miserable. A couple of years ago, Ida moved to Florida to be with her daughter, a former teacher who is in her early seventies. Shortly after moving to Florida, Ida threw her walker away and now stands upright and walks without any aid at all! How did she attain this miracle? She started working out with her daughter!

A typical Monday for Ida now begins at Sun City Fitness Center at about eleven a.m. like this: **stretching on the ballet barre; arm extensions; a two-mile walk on the treadmill; walking up and down a group of steps; twenty minutes on the row machine; leg presses on a weight machine; and finally, bicep curls with fifty-eight pounds of weight.** Whew! I'm glad that I don't work out there; Ida would show me up! Her workout is more intense than mine! Not only that, but after working out on her birthday last year, she partied at the gym! So, if you're over one hundred years old and tell me that you're too old, I still won't believe you! You are never too old, and it's never too late! Ida's daughter deserves much of the credit; she motivated Ida to get working, largely due to the fact that she couldn't lift her anymore! Ida began small, working out to a television program called *Sit to Be fit*. Soon Ida was able to do the exercises standing up, and there was no stopping her after that!

I first learned of Ida Wasserman from the *Tampa Tribune* (1/29/08), a newspaper that I read when I was living in Florida. I couldn't believe it myself! Ida has served as an inspiration to many people, including those in her own family. Her oldest son, Ed, is seventy-five years old, and Ida constantly gets on him about working out! Wasserman also has brothers and sisters, two sets of twins, eighty-seven and ninety, and they're still going strong as well. In addition to throwing away her walker, Ida is also not hunched over any longer! She is truly an inspiration to anyone who has the wrong kind of mentality about fitness! If you find yourself with any kind of physical problem, let Ida Wasserman inspire you too. Life begins at one hundred; just ask anyone who knows Ida Wasserman.

Now, having looked at the amazing story of Ida Wasserman, I want you to be inspired but at the same time realistic! If you are over forty, then you have to exercise great care in choosing a physical fitness program that's right for you. Each year that goes by brings about greater challenges, but you can still see good results in a fitness program that is designed for you as an individual! And of course, the greater the challenge becomes, the more important it is to get into a fitness program, even if you are at your target weight! The proof of that can be seen in **AARP magazine's July and August** 2007 issue. They note that two studies that analyzed the effects of strength training in adults between the ages of fifty and seventy saw a 10–15 percent decrease in belly fat despite no weight loss. Just because you aren't overweight doesn't necessarily mean that you aren't out of shape! Fat weighs less than muscle, which means that you can get into shape, lose the belly fat, and not change what you weigh! The same magazine notes that several studies were done to show that people who were at their target weight still lost belly fat when they began a workout program and their muscle tone increased! Get with a program today! Your age doesn't matter.

America is an aging country. Statistics show that in 1900, about 4 percent of the population was over eighty-five years old; today the number is over 10 percent and is still growing. Between 1900 and 1990, human life expectancy has grown by about twenty-seven years. This means that more and more, people who begin a training program are over forty. Hormone levels change as we age, and that makes it more difficult to lose the weight.

Many over forty who do not lower their caloric intake will gain a middle age spread. Most people in that age group will consume the same amount of calories, and their level of activity decreases. It is estimated that your caloric intake should go down by about a hundred calories per year for each year after you turn forty. This will help you maintain optimum weight. We, of course, either don't know or don't care about these things as a society, and that is why we let ourselves go! Those who care about what is happening to their bodies will do something about it!

We have already discussed earlier that we lose muscle mass as we grow older. This loss of muscle mass leads to muscle imbalances, which causes shoulders to slump forward and other misshaping of the body. These imbalances can lead to loss of range of motion, loss of balance, and the limited mobility seen in older adults. This loss of muscle mass also leads to lower metabolism, which helps to increase the body fat that we accumulate as we age! The decrease in muscle mass also helps to explain why we start to lose stability and balance as strength in the stabilizer muscles decreases. This will mean that as you enter a fitness program you will have to concentrate more on balance exercises than a younger individual does.

As you age, you must approach the fitness program differently than your younger counterpart does. This includes the nutrition part of the program as well! It is important that you take in more protein than your younger counterpart does, due to the slowing of the metabolism. If you do not take in enough protein, then your body will break down your muscle mass to use the proper protein for maintaining the function of your organs.

As we saw in the chapter on nutrition, we should not eat three big meals per day but rather several small ones! This is even truer among older adults. Every time you eat, take in some form of protein—poultry, fish, eggs, nuts, nut butters, and protein supplements. Use low-fat and nonfat dairy products.

When you begin a fitness program, start slowly! **You should begin with these steps: <u>Touch your toes and see how far down you can reach.</u>** This will determine flexibility. **<u>Stand on one foot.</u>** This will determine your balance. **Seated chest press,** one set; **Seated cable row,** one set; **Leg press or Squat,** one set; **Stationary bike or Treadmill,** one set. This or something like it should be your first workout session. If a trainer tries to get you to do too much, don't be afraid to let him/ her know that you are being over-exerted. If a trainer is young, he or she may not have had an older client before. If you approach your workout correctly, soon you will be doing as much or more than some of your younger counterparts, but once again, and I cannot stress this enough, the older you are, the more caution you should take at the beginning of your training program, especially if you have not been active for years! **Establish a baseline.** Do not be too overzealous in your determination to get into shape. Depending on your age and fitness level, you will probably have experienced considerable loss in joint integrity, flexibility, and range of motion. Continued workouts may help restore some of these conditions.

Focus on upper body movements. This will help restore the core and spine, which will improve posture. **Stretching.** This should be cautiously included to maximize range of flexibility Use the treadmill sparingly: Anything that will aggravate the joints at the impact of the foot can cause back problems.

There is a lot more that can go wrong with an older client. That of course doesn't mean that you should ignore a healthy workout; just proceed with caution!

When you begin a workout regimen as an older person, you have to remember that your body is not the same as it used to be. Our bones become smaller, our skin starts to lose its elasticity and will begin to sag, and our cardiovascular health begins to decline. Our hormone levels begin to lower, and that affects our ability to increase muscle size. We have to take care not to work out the same way as our younger counterparts in the gym! If we injure ourselves, then it will take longer for us to recover!

As we get older, we are also more prone to high blood pressure, which is another reason to get into a fitness program, because exercise helps us to control our blood pressure. Controlling our blood pressure helps to reduce the instances of stroke and kidney disease.

Your range of motion will be more limited because of degeneration of the connective tissue in the joints. You may not be able to do something simple, like fully extending your arms over your head, at least not at first! The more you exercise the more you will fight the effects of aging! Of course, you will never be eighteen again, but you can regain some of the motion and posture that you lost as you started to age! Let's look at individuals who have successfully combated aging, just like Ida Wassermann: **Jake Lalanne**, the most popular name in modern fitness. He is definitely an inspiration to all ages. Mr. Lalanne is the first trainer to bring exercise programs to television. Jack is now in his nineties, but he looks about fifty! According to his web site, www.jacklalanne.com, Jack wasn't always into fitness! But now he is "the Godfather of Fitness." From his web site:

JACK LALANNE FEATS:

1954 Age 40: Swam the length of the San Francisco Golden Gate Bridge underwater with 140 pounds of equipment, including two air tanks … an undisputed world record. **1955** Age 41: Swam, handcuffed, from Alcatraz to Fisherman's Wharf in San Francisco, CA. **1956** Age 42: Set a world record of 1,033 pushups in 23 minutes on *You Asked for It*, a TV Show with Art Baker. **1957** Age 43: Swam the treacherous Golden Gate Channel, towing a 2,500-pound cabin cruiser. This involved fighting the cold, swift ocean currents that made the 1 mile swim a 6 ½ mile test of strength and endurance. **1958** Age 44: Maneuvered a paddleboard 30 miles, 9 ½ hours non-stop from Farallon Islands to the San Francisco shore. **1959** Age 45: Completed 1,000 pushups and 1,000 chin-ups in 1 hour and 22 minutes. "Happy" is born and *The Jack Lalanne Show* goes nationwide. **1974** Age 60: Swam from Alcatraz Island to Fisherman's Wharf, for a second time, handcuffed, shackled, and towing a 1,000-pound boat. **1975** Age 61: Swam the length of the Golden Gate Bridge, underwater, for a second time handcuffed, shackled and towing a 1,000-pound boat. **1976** Age 62: Commemorating the "Spirit of '76," swam 1 mile in Long Beach Harbor, handcuffed, shackled, and towing 13 boats (representing the 13 original colonies) containing 76 people. **1979** Age 65: Towed 65 boats filled with 6,500-pounds of Louisiana Pacific wood pulp while handcuffed and shackled in Lake Ashinoko, near Tokyo, Japan. **1980** Age 66: Towed 10 boats in North Miami, Florida filled with 77 people for over a mile in less than 1 hour. **1984** Age 70: Handcuffed, shackled and fighting strong winds and currents, towed 70 boats with 70 people from the Queen's Way Bridge in the Long Beach Harbor to the Queen Mary, 1 ½ miles. **1992** Age 78: Academy of Body Building and Fitness Award. **1994** Age 80: State of California Governor's Council on Physical Fitness Lifetime Achievement Award. **1996** Age 82: Dwight D. Eisenhower Fitness Award. **1999** Age 85: Spirit of Muscle Beach Award. **2002** Age 88: Jack receives his very own star on the Hollywood Blvd. Walk of Fame. **2004** Age 90: Jack celebrates his birthday with a major media blitz in New York, San Francisco, and Los Angeles. ESPN Classic runs a 24-hour marathon of the original Jack Lalanne Shows. **2005** Age 91: Received the Jack Webb Award from the Los Angeles Police Historical Society, the Arnold Classic Lifetime Achievement Award, Interglobal's International Infomercial Award, the Freddie, Medical Media Public Service Award. Jack Lalanne's birth date is Sep. 26, 1914.

Arnold Alois Schwarzenegger: Arnold is now in his sixties! But as anyone who has seen *Terminator Three* can attest to, he is in as good shape now as he was in his twenties! From bodybuilding to acting and politics, he has succeeded where many would not have even tried! Arnold would be active in sports from the time he was thirteen and decided on bodybuilding as a career at fifteen! His first movie was *Hercules in New York,* playing the same character as two of his idols: Steve Reeves and Reg Park. Thus, from 1970 to 2004, Schwarzenegger has been a top box office draw until he entered the political world when he was elected governor (R) of California. He is married to Maria Shriver.

Lou Jude Ferrigno: Lou Ferrigno is television's "Incredible Hulk" to Bill Bixby's David Banner. He, at age fifty-six, is in as good a shape now as he was back when he was on "The Incredible Hulk" (1978–82). He has appeared in both Hulk feature films as a security guard. (In fact, he is the only actor to appear in both "Hulk" films.) Lou Ferrigno suffered an ear infection that took away 80 percent of his hearing! He cites this incident along with the verbal abuse connected with it as the reason he got into bodybuilding.

Ferrigno also cites Steve Reeves as one of his idols, just like Arnold Schwarzenegger, and like Schwarzenegger, also played Hercules in a couple of low-budget Italian films. Lou would compete with Schwarzenegger at many bodybuilding events but never defeat him. He would beat out Schwarzenegger one time, however, when he gained the role of television's "Incredible Hulk" simply because he was taller than his Australian rival.

Sylvester Gardenzio Stallone: At the age of sixty-two, Stallone is still going strong! He has been in six successful *Rocky* films and four installments of *Rambo*. He was born in 1946 and had suffered a birth defect that resulted in partial paralysis of his face, which is why his lip droops and his speech is slurred. Stallone's first film appearance was in the Woody Allen film *Bananas*. Unlike Schwarzenegger and Ferrigno, Stallone would lose his shape for a time, and it was during this time that he appeared in one of his most critically acclaimed roles, in *Copland*. Robert De Niro's character even referred to Stallone's character as a "creampuff." Stallone would come roaring back into shape, however, and reprise his roles of "Rocky" and "Rambo" one more time in 2006.

Others who have stayed in shape and are still doing immensely well include Harrison Ford, Ron Perlman, and Pierce Brosnan.

With inspiration like this, how can you tell me, or yourself, that you are too old to get into shape? You are never too old! Get to the gym and see those results! A popular hip-hop song states: "Age ain't nuthin' but a number!" Ida Wasserman, Jack Lalanne, Arnold Schwarzenegger, Lou Ferrigno, Sylvester Stallone, Harrison Ford, Ron Perlman, and many more are living proof that there is no such thing as a middle age spread!

Counting Calories:
Here is a basic calorie guide to start you on a proper nutrition program!

Fruit   Cals

Apple (5oz/150g) 60
Apricot (Dried or Fresh) 10
Avocado 230
Banana (4oz/115g) 70
Banana chips (per oz/28g) 145
Berries (1oz/28g) 8
Canned fruit in own juice (1oz/28g) 10
Cherries (4oz/115g) 44
Clementines/Tangerines 25
Coconut (1oz/28g) 99
Currants (1oz/28g) 75
Dates (Dried or Fresh) 15
Grapefruit (half) 40
Grapes (4oz/115g) 68
Kiwi 35
Lemon/Lime 19/3
Mandarins (canned in juice, 4oz/115g) 40
Mango 110
Melon (1 wedge) 30
Nectarine (6oz/175g) 60
Orange 60
Passion Fruit 5
Peach (6oz/175g) 50
Pear (6oz/175g) 60
Pineapple (1oz/28g) 12
Pineapple ring 20
Plum 10
Prune 10
Star Fruit (each) 50

Vegetables

Beet root 10
Broccoli (boiled) 7
Cabbage (boiled) 5
Carrots (boiled) 7
Cauliflower (boiled) 8
Celery 2
Cucumber 3
Leek (boiled) 6
Lettuce 4
Mushroom 4
Onion rings (in breadcrumbs or batter) 30
Onion, spring 2
Onions 20
Parsnip (boiled/roast) 19/30
Peas, dried (boiled) 31
Peas, fresh/frozen 19
Peas, garden (canned) 23
Peas, processed (canned) 28
Peppers (green) 24
Peppers (orange, red, or yellow) 50
Potato 21
Potato, sweet 24
Sweet corn (baby) 7
Sweet corn (canned) 35
Tomatoes (canned/fresh) 5
Tomatoes (sun-dried) 42
Turnips (boiled) 4
Water chestnuts (canned) 9
Watercress 6

Fish:

Uncooked (per oz/28g)
Cod (fillet) 22
Cod (in batter-oven baked) 59
Cod (in parsley sauce) 24
Crab (in brine) 22
Fish finger 44

Haddock (fillet) 21
Haddock (in batter) 65
Haddock (in crumbs) 49
Hake (fillet) 20
Herring (fillet) 56
Kippers (fillet) 75
Mackerel (fillet) 63
Mackerel (smoked) 99
Oysters (each) 7
Salmon 52
Salmon, pink (in brine) 43
Salmon, red (in brine) 47
Sardines (in brine) 48
Sardines (in tomato sauce) 45
Sardines (raw) 55
Scampi (in breadcrumbs) 60
Scampi (raw) 30
Trout (fillet) 39
Tuna (fresh) 44
Tuna (in brine/water) 22
Tuna (in oil) 53

Chicken

Cals per 10 oz/28g
Breast, casseroled 32
Breast, meat only, grilled 41
Dark meat, roasted 55
Leg, meat and skin, roasted 66
Chicken Minced, raw 55 3calories
Roasted 50

Turkey

Dark meat, roasted 50 1.9
Light meat, roasted 55 3.6

Duck

Meat only, roasted 55 2.9

Beef

Brisket, lean, boiled 63 3.1
Fillet steak, grilled   53 2.2
Minced, raw 63 4.5
Roast beef 50 1.7
Rump steak, lean, grilled 50 1.7
Sirloin, lean, grilled 63 2.8
Sirloin, lean, roasted 53 1.8
Topside, lean, roasted   57 1.8

Lamb

Belly joint, grilled 90 6.6
Breast, lean, roasted 76 5.2
Leg, lean, roasted 57 2.6
Leg chops, lean, grilled 62 3.4
Loin chops, lean, grilled 69 5

Pork

Diced, lean, casseroled 52 1.8
Fillet, lean & fat, raw 41 1.8
Leg joint, lean, roasted 52 1.4
Loin chop, lean, grilled 221 7.7
Minced, raw 46 2.7
Spare ribs, lean, grilled 37 2.5
Steaks, lean, grilled 55 2.1

Cheese

Blue Stilton   102 8.8
Brie 91 8.0
Cheddar 8.6 1.5
Cheddar 1/2 fat 65 3.9
Cheese (spread) 8.6 5.8
Cream Cheese, Extra Light   30 1.2
Cream Cheese, Low Fat 47 3.7
Edam 93 7.1
Edam ½ fat 71 3.2
Feta 76 6.2
Low-Fat Cottage Cheese 20 0.4

Bread

Cals per oz 28g

Bagel (small/large) 160/225 0.9/1.3

Baguette (small/large) 250/400 1.0/1.8

Bread stick 20 0.1

Croissant, large 295 17.5

Fat French 77 0.8

Garlic Bread 100 5.7

Hamburger bun small/large 155/225 3.4/4.3

Muffin 150 1.3

Pita Bread White (small/large) 180/90 2.2/1

Rye 63 0.5

Soda Bread 75 0.7

White, sliced 67 0.5

Whole meal/Wheat/Brown 61 0.7

ABOUT THE AUTHOR:

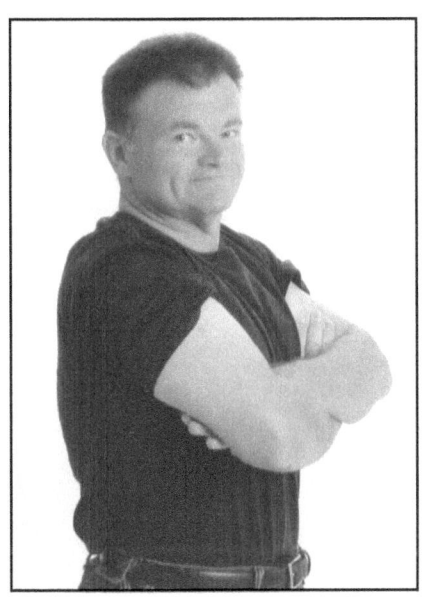

Kevin given is a personal trainer with the Private Trainers Association. He has lost over sixty pounds with the help of a personal trainer, and he has become a trainer in an effort to show others how they can succeed in achieving physical fitness and personal wellness. Kevin has been in radio since he was fourteen years old, working as a DJ in Maine, Florida, and California. He produced and hosted the radio program *Legends of Rock*, which was heard worldwide on the web through KCLA. com radio. Kevin was born in Houlton, Maine, moved to Largo, Florida, in 1996, and now resides in Torrance, California. This is his first book.

RECOMMENDED READING:

Fitness Nutrition for Special Dietary Needs, Stella Lucia Volpe

Strength Training Anatomy, Frederick Delavier

Body Building Anatomy, Nick Evans

Muscle Mechanics, Everett Aaberg

Women's Strength Training Anatomy, Frederick Delavier

Strength Training for Women, Lori Incledon

Smart Drugs and Nutrition, Ward Dean, M.D.

Smart Drugs 2, Ward Dean, M.D.

Power Lifting, Frederick C. Hatfield

Bill Pearls Keys to Inner Universe, Bill Pearl

Exercise Physiology, William D. McArdle, Frank I. Katch and Victor L. Katch

All books are available on the web at www.propta.com.

WEIGHT LOSS AND FITNESS PERIODICALS INCLUDE:
+ **Muscle and Fitness**

+ *Flex*

  Offering inside info about the bodybuilding world, including news, photos, and information about training and nutrition.

+ *Iron Man Magazine*

  Iron Man Magazine is an open forum on bodybuilding that inspires, informs, entertains, and promotes this discipline's power to develop the mind and body into an integrated whole.

+ *Muscle Media*

  Muscle, fitness, nutrition, supplement, and steroid information.

+ *Real Solutions Magazine*

  Weight training, muscle building, and fitness magazine.

+ *Hardgainer*

  Provides common sense information on bodybuilding and weight training.

+ *Natural Muscle Magazine*

  Publication covering drug-free bodybuilding and fitness.

+ *Muscular Development*

  Provides the latest information on strength training, bodybuilding, nutrition, fitness, and health.

+ *Robert Kennedy's MuscleMag International*

  Offers articles, photos, and more.

+ The Exercise Group

  Publishers of *Natural Bodybuilding & Fitness*, *Exercise for Men Only*, and *Men's Exercise*.

+ *Testosterone: Muscle With Attitude*

Physique publication for hardcore muscle building.

+ *Master Trainer*
Training advice and personal training for weightlifters and bodybuilders dedicated to lifetime fitness.

+ *Hardcore Muscle*
Focusing on training, lifestyle, attitude, bodybuilders, and babes.

+ *Anabolic Insider*
Covers anabolic steroids, cutting-edge supplements, specialized training techniques, and nutrition articles.

+ *Thorax's Iron Magazine*
Wide range of information for bodybuilders.

+ *Mind and Muscle Magazine*
Featuring articles about nutrition, training, bodybuilding.

+ *MuscleZine*
Includes articles from top fitness professionals, chat, and forum section.

+ *FLEX magazine*
Interactive bodybuilding resource from Australia.

+ *Muscle Maker*
Myogenic, lipotropic, and ergogenic truth.

+ *Flex Europe*
Bodybuilding resource containing news, events, and competition results. Complete with expert advice.

www.ingramcontent.com/pod-product-compliance
Lightning Source LLC
Chambersburg PA
CBHW021258280526
45784CB00005B/2417